Water Aerobic Ex
Made Easy for Seniors
and Everyone

A Comprehensive Step-By-Step Guide to Water Aerobics for Full Body Workout For Seniors and Everyone Including Those with Mobility Impairment

Introduction

Who doesn't want to spend their senior years lounging, laughing with friends and family, and enjoying activities they love? For many of us, that's the life we dream of and aspire to. But as the years go by, the realization sinks in that we are no longer as young as we used to be and that this plays a role in how far we can push our bodies when engaging in exercise or physical activity.

This realization can be disheartening.

But with that realization comes the opportunity to exercise in water. Water exercises have all the benefits of exercises done on land minus the aches and pains. Before long, you'll be able to enjoy various physical activities as your body regains its strength and flexibility and say goodbye to the varied symptoms associated with growing older.

So:

Don't suffer in silence. Instead, embrace water exercises and get a full body workout.

Dig in to get started!

PS: I'd like your feedback. If you are happy with this book, please leave a review on Amazon.

Please leave a review for this book on Amazon by visiting the page below:

https://amzn.to/2VMR5qr

Table of Content

Chapter 1: Getting Started With Water Aerobics

Exercising in water sounds more fun than exercising on land. But you mustn't forget that you will still be stretching your body, burning calories, and giving yourself a full body workout. These are things you should not do lightly.

You need to plan.

Fundamentally, three important questions can help you prepare. These include:

What Benefits Can I Get From Doing Water Exercises?

Before you jump into the water, you need to learn why you need to embrace water exercises in the first place. This will help you stick to a schedule and motivate you to continue your new exercise routine.

The benefits of water exercises include:

Improves heart health

Water aerobics is a low-impact workout; yes, but make no mistake, it will still increase your heart rate. It helps you work out your heart muscles and does an impressive job of improving circulation, making it an effective way to improve the heart health[1] of people suffering from heart issues such as coronary heart disease.

The hydrostatic pressure of water provides the needed resistance to get your heart pumping, thus reducing the risk of heart disease. And as time goes by, you can use weights to increase the intensity of your workout and improve your heart health.

Enhances balance and coordination

One symptom of aging is reduced coordination. That is why you must work on improving your balance and physical control.

Water gives you a safer environment in which to exercise. Unlike exercising on land, you won't fall when you exercise in water. Rather, if you make a mistake, you'll float, regain your balance and continue exercising. You can work on controlling a wide range of movements. Moreover, studies[23] show that

---

[1]

https://www.sciencedirect.com/science/article/pii/S1836955321000928

[2] https://www.ncbi.nlm.nih.gov/pmc/articles/PMC3781896/

[3] https://bmcgeriatr.biomedcentral.com/articles/10.1186/1471-2318-8-19

water can improve your balance and coordination. And as your control improves, you'll see the results even as you walk on land.

Easy on the joints

Two main things make it easier for you to exercise in water. The first thing is water buoyancy. This characteristic is useful in supporting your body weight as you exercise. The second thing is the impact of water on gravity. When you exercise in a pool, water helps you mitigate the negative impact of gravity on your ankles, knees, hips, and back.

Thus, when you engage in water exercises, it cushions your joints, tendons, and ligaments from damage. Water also relieves pain[4], a bonus if you experience aches and pains—as is usually the case with most seniors.

If you suffer from diseases such as arthritis or other muscle conditions, you will benefit greatly from exercising in water. Since water supports various movements, you'll be able to increase your strength, build endurance and improve flexibility and general fitness.

---

[4] https://www.ncbi.nlm.nih.gov/pmc/articles/PMC3781896/

Reduces risk of injury

Bone fragility and lowered balance are the core things that increase a senior's risk of falling, especially when exercising. For some, this increased risk of falling is enough to stop them from exercising. Fortunately, water aerobics reduces this risk due to the supportive nature of water.

When you exercise in water, the balance loss won't have the same impact as it would on land. This expands the range of exercises you can perform without the risk of injury.

Enhances weight loss

Your weight can increase or reduce the burden of disease. As such, it is important to engage in water aerobics to maintain a healthy body weight.

Water aerobics burn calories[5]. Remember that water provides more resistance than air. Thus, the same exercises you do on land will often enable you to burn more calories if you perform them on water.

But more than that, water exercises help you strengthen your body and build muscle mass. That is important since the loss

---

[5] https://www.ncbi.nlm.nih.gov/pmc/articles/PMC4106774/

of muscle mass becomes more pronounced as you grow older. If you work to build your muscle mass, your body will thank you as you enter your senior years.

All in all, the restorative nature of water is something you need to take advantage of, whether you are a senior or not. Water heals, yes, but it also helps prevent health issues, which is very good.

Let's now look at the next question you need to ask yourself before you engage in water aerobics.

What Equipment Do I Need For Aerobic Exercises?

You don't need special equipment to perform water exercises. However, a few things can come in handy when you're exercising.

These include:

A towel

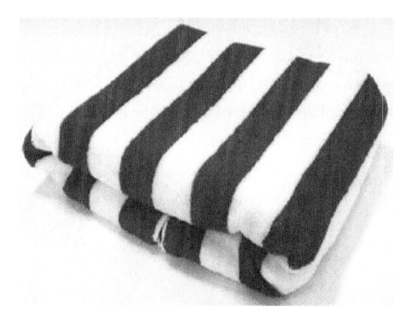

A towel or two will be handy before and after you complete your exercises.

A swim cap

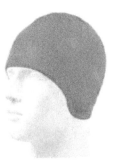

If you're planning to use a swimming cap, you should ensure that it fits you comfortably. If you have long hair, you should ensure that your hair can fit into the cap if you do not want to expose it to chemicals and risk damaging it.

A pair of goggles

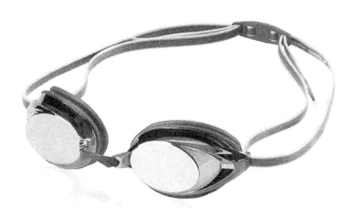

If you're uncomfortable with water getting into your eyes as you perform water aerobics, you should invest in a pair of goggles.

Kickboard

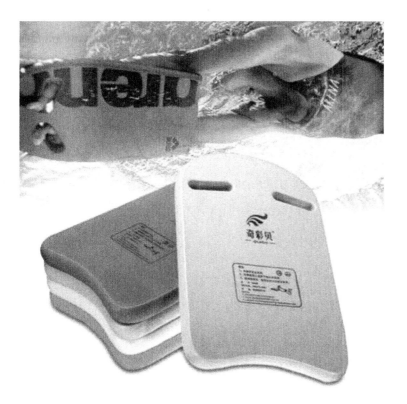

When you're doing water exercises, you may want some extra support. A kickboard will help you stay afloat. You can hold on to it as you do lower body exercises.

Foam dumbbells

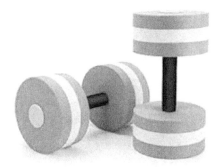

Foam dumbbells are deceptive in that they are lightweight when dry. However, once you place them in water, they become heavier. You can use them to add resistance as you exercise.

Try holding the foam dumbbells in your hands before purchasing since you may have to hold them for a while as you exercise. Buy the ones that feel comfortable to hold.

Resistance gloves and hand paddles

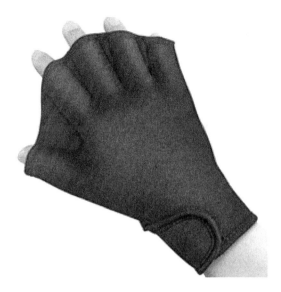

These products are great for those who want to boost their strength training. They will make your hands heavier and help you exercise your arm and shoulder muscles.

Wrist and ankle weights

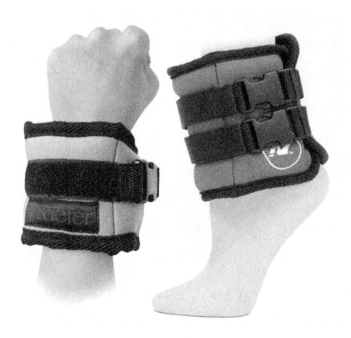

As you become more comfortable with exercising, you may want to increase the intensity of the exercises. You can do this by using ankle and wrist weights. They will look increase resistance as you work out in the water.

Buoyancy belt

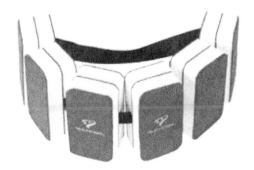

A buoyancy belt does an excellent job at keeping you afloat as you do arm exercises.

As with any equipment, please familiarize yourself with whatever equipment you plan to use because it will keep you safe and help you get the most out of the equipment. But even with the right equipment, you still need to follow some rules to keep safe when you're in the water.

What Safety Tips Should I Consider When Doing Aerobic Exercises?

The first thing you should do before engaging in water aerobics is to talk to your doctor. This is especially important if you are taking medication or recovering from an injury. Your doctor will advise you on what to do to exercise safely.

But there are other things you should also do. You should:

Familiarize yourself with the pool

You need to familiarize yourself with the facilities you'll be using before you start exercising. If you're using public facilities, go for a tour and ask questions to get a better feel of the location. Also, ensure you know the location of the stairs and ladders of the pool and the depth of water.

Furthermore, it would be good to know any in-place pool rules or policies meant to safeguard everyone. You should also know important dates when the pool won't be available so you can plan accordingly.

Exercise with a partner

No one wants to think of getting into an accident when using the pool. Unfortunately, bad things can happen when you least expect them. That is why it is important to exercise with a partner.

A trainer, a lifeguard, or a friend can watch over you as you exercise. If you're exercising as a group, you can have one person keep an eye on you even as you keep an eye on them.

A partner can act as your cheerleader and a competitor. When you think of quitting, your partner can give you a pep talk to remind you why you need to tough it out until things get better.

Stick to the shallow end

While you may want to head straight to the deep end, this is not advisable. Remember, you are here to exercise, not to showcase your swimming skills. Even if you're a professional swimmer, you will benefit from exercising at the shallow end because if you need a break, you can take it without treading water.

Pace yourself

Time tends to go by faster when you're in the pool. But you shouldn't overdo it. You need to set a timer and get out of the pool once done with the exercises. Plan to exercise for about 30 to 45 minutes, 3 to 5 days a week. If you feel like you can still go on, it would be best to increase the intensity of the exercise rather than the time you spend in the pool.

Remember, you are not competing with anyone. Rather, you are exercising to improve your health and well-being. As such, it is important to take precautions and pace yourself to ensure you can get positive results as you engage in a full-body workout

But what type of water exercises should you engage in?

Let's discuss this in the next chapter.

Chapter 2: Water Walking and Jogging Exercises

Walking, jogging, and running are some of the most common low-impact aerobic exercises doable in the comfort of a pool or another body of water. Such exercises boost strength and endurance and improve mobility. But more than that, they promote cardiovascular health, a quality that is vital to any aerobic activity.

Best of all, people of all ages and varying levels of fitness can perform the exercises.

Let's take a closer look at the exercises:

Regular water walking

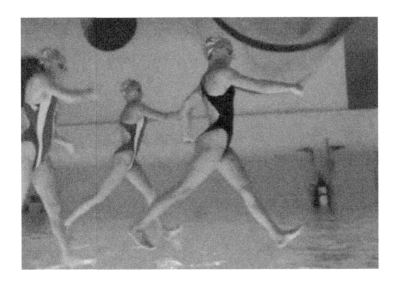

If you love going for walks, you'll no doubt be interested in water walking, especially if you want to increase the benefits of walking.

As you already know, water provides added resistance, increasing your workout's intensity. If you walk in a pool, your whole body will be involved as you walk since it will be submerged in water and facing resistance.

To perform this exercise, you need to:

1. Step into the pool and ensure the water covers most of your body.

2. Stand up straight. Your back and shoulders should be straight, and your arms should be by your sides.

3. Look straight ahead as you engage your core, and then take a long stride. Your walking stride should be a bit longer than the one you would normally take on land, but it should not make you feel uncomfortable.

4. As your right foot hits the ground, swing your left arm and then swing your right arm as the left foot hits the ground.

5. Place one foot in front of the other until you reach the other side of the pool, then turn and continue with the exercise.

6. If you're not used to walking in a pool, start slowly by walking for 5 to 25 minutes. Use a timer to time your workout and concentrate on your hand and leg movements. Also, remember to turn slowly to keep your balance as you walk back to the starting point.

If you can reach your target, you should endeavor to exercise up to 5 days a week and then gradually increase the time you exercise. Next, work on increasing your walking speed. This way, your exercise time won't change, but the intensity of the exercise will increase.

Another thing you can do is use resistance gloves, wrist and ankle weights, or a pair of dumbbells to increase the level of difficulty of your workouts.

As always, make gradual changes and cut back on your exercise time if need be so that your body can adjust to the increased intensity.

Sideways water walking

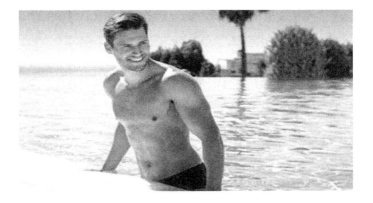

Sideways water walking is an exercise specifically designed to target your inner and outer thighs even as it exercises the rest of your body. You'll essentially be taking steps to your sides. The movements involved will help you improve your balance and spatial awareness. You'll also be able to improve your flexibility and engage a lot of your muscles.

To perform this exercise, you should:

1. Stand inside the pool with your back straight and your arms positioned at your sides.

2. Move your right hip to your side, and then move your right foot. As you perform this exercise, your hip should always lead before you take a step to the side. Do not lead with your foot.

3. Next, lift your left foot off the ground and move it towards your right foot. Continue taking side steps until you reach the end of the swimming pool.

4. Once you reach the end, move your left foot to the side. Don't forget to lead with your left hip.

5. Next, lift your right foot off the ground and bring it towards your left foot. Continue with the same formation until you reach your target.

As you would do with regular water walking, you can also set a timer for sideways water walking. Start slow and gradually increase the walk's pace, time, and intensity. If you find placing your arms by your sides uncomfortable, you can clasp them gently at your chest area as you exercise.

Sideways water walking changes the way you usually walk. As such, it may burden your body more than you expect. Take your time and ensure there are no red flags before you continue with the exercise. If you'd like, you can use a kickboard for added support as you start the exercise. But with time, you should get rid of the kickboard and add some weights to your exercise routine.

Also, it is best to check your neck movements as you walk. Normally, people live seeing where they step, but abruptly turning your neck to your side as you walk is not advisable. Instead, keep your eyes in front of you and judge the distance by looking through the periphery instead of repeatedly turning to check.

Jogging and running

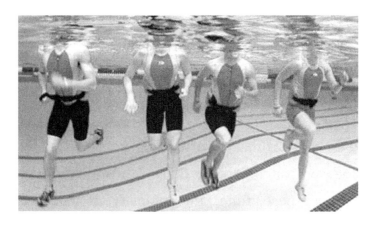

Water jogging and running increase the intensity of water exercises as they require you to bend various body parts, increase your pace and burn more calories than regular water walking.

However, since you'll be running in water, the running you end up doing may differ from conventional running because, depending on where you exercise, your feet may not be able to touch the ground.

To engage in water jogging or running, you should:

1. Enter the pool and determine your exercise position.

2. Next, you need to stand upright and then start jogging. Lift your right leg up and forward as you move your left hand forward, and then lift your left leg up and forward as you move your right hand forward. Your upper body should lean slightly forward as you jog.

3. Breathe deeply as you jog and jog for 3 to 5 minutes. If you're planning to run instead of jog, run for 3 to 5 minutes at an increased pace.

Ideally, you'll want to jog or run with your body submerged in water. This may require you to 'cycle' as you move your legs. Breathe deeply as you engage in the exercise, and use a floatation device if necessary.

Water marching

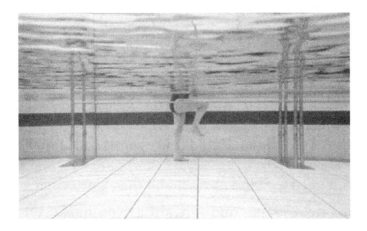

Water marching is another exercise you can use when you want to increase resistance. However, be mindful enough to maintain a rhythmic march instead of switching up the pace now and then.

To match in a pool, you should:

1. Stand up straight in an area of the pool where the water level is just at your hip level.

2. Start matching as you lift your leg to your knees and swing your hands. Keep your toes pointing forward.

3. Match for about 2 to 3 minutes.

4. As you become more comfortable with matching, you can increase the intensity of the exercise by moving your arms and legs more energetically.

When walking in a swimming pool, you can walk slowly before and after your workout to stretch your body. Walk for at least five minutes and start your water walking workout or stretch your body before entering the pool, especially if you're planning to exercise in a cool pool.

As you can see, there are several variations of exercises you can use when you want to perform water walking. However, it is good to note that while water walking falls in the full-body workout category, you need to up your exercise routine if you really want to exercise your whole body.

Water exercises are great for beginners or those who want to spice up their exercise routine between other exercises. But there are other aerobic exercises you should perform to engage your full body.

Let's take a look at them.

Chapter 3: Water Exercises For Cardio

Cardio pool exercises increase your heart rate and allow you to exercise your whole body. For best results, try to do each of the following exercises ten times and repeat the exercise circuit 3 times.

The exercises include:

Water walking

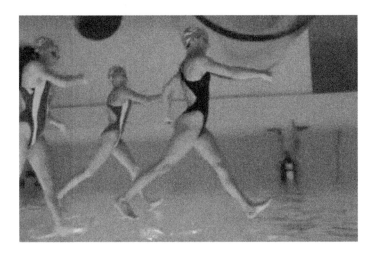

Please do this exercise in the shallow end:

1. Stand up straight at one shallow end and face the other end of the shallow end.

2. Proceed to walk at a comfortable pace towards the other side as your hands move naturally in tune with your steps.

3. Once you reach the shallow end, turn around and return to the starting point.

4. Repeat the exercise up to 10 times.

Remember to keep your arms under the water as you walk. This will allow you to work your arm and shoulder muscles. If you're comfortable in the pool, you should exercise in chest-deep water. But you can exercise in waist-deep water if you don't know how to swim. Either way, allow your arms to touch the water for added resistance.

Knee kicks

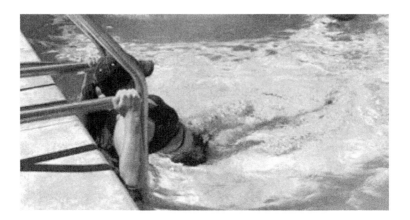

To do this exercise, your should:

1. Move to the pool's side and rest your back and arms on it.

2. Next, bring your right knee up and pull your leg in before kicking it straight out and back down.

3. Bring your left knee up and pull your left leg in before kicking it straight out and back down.

4. Alternate the leg kicks and repeat the exercise 10 times.

5. Repeat the exercise circuit 3 times.

Knee kicks are a lower body exercise, but they will still get your heart pumping.

As you can imagine, you'll need a good sense of balance if you want to perform this exercise with proper form. That is why it is important to support your back.

However, it is possible to do the exercise by holding on to a pool noodle. Keep your back straight and stick to the shallow end so your leg can have a solid place to land as you bring it back down.

Frog kicks

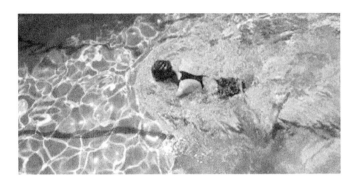

To perform this exercise, you should:

1. Stand up straight, facing the wall, then stretch your hands to hold onto the pool wall. If you have a pool noodle, you can grip it instead of holding the wall.

2. Allow your lower body to float behind you, then pull your legs in. Your knees should bend out as if you're trying to make your legs move towards your lower back.

3. Kick each leg straight out as if you're trying to make a triangle with your lower body, and then return the legs to the center.

4. Repeat the frog kicks ten times.

5. Do three circuits of the exercises.

The trick to doing frog kicks is to get a good grip on your pool noodle or firmly grip the wall. This way, you won't break the rhythm of the kicks as you exercise.

Bicep curls

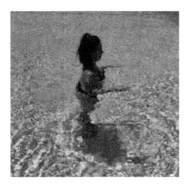

Bicep curls are great for stretching your upper body. To perform this exercise, you need to:

1. Find a comfortable place you can stand in. Ideally, the water should be chest deep since you want to exercise your upper body, but you can exercise in waist-deep water if you wish.

2. Place your hands at your sides and proceed to open your palms.

3. Turn your hands such that your palms face to the front with your arms still by your sides. Proceed to squeeze your fingers against each other. You may feel a little stretch when you press your fingers together.

4. Bend your elbows and move your hands towards your shoulders. Your fingertips should curl in to touch your

shoulders; do your best to keep your upper arms at your sides as you do the exercise.

5. Move your arms back down and return them to your sides.

6. Repeat the exercise 10 times.

7. Do three circuits of the exercises.

Your biceps play an important role when it comes to supporting your forearm. They allow you to lift, lower and rotate your forearms; thus, you must exercise them to avoid straining your muscles.

But even as you exercise your biceps, you must take care not to overdo it. It would be better to do fewer circuits of the exercise instead of trying to make your biceps stronger overnight. If you are patient, you will gradually strengthen your muscles, which will allow you to lift various things without aches and pains.

Triceps extension

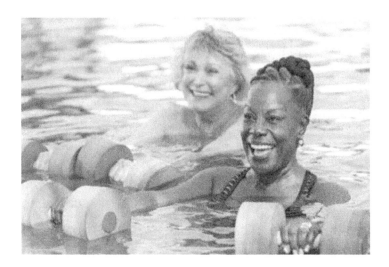

As with your biceps, your triceps are also useful when you want to perform the pushing and pulling function. That is why you need to exercise your upper arms even as you exercise your lower arms. Exercising both your biceps and triceps will improve your functional movement and greatly reduce the risk of injury as you carry things.

To exercise your triceps, you should:

1. Stand up straight inside the pool and press both of your elbows towards your sides.

2. Make a 90-degree angle by bending your elbows. Your hands should be out and in front of you. Both your forearms should be parallel to the ground.

3. Move your arms backward and quickly stretch your lower arms behind you as you stretch your triceps.

4. Return your arms to the 90-degree position in front of you.

5. Repeat the exercise 10 times.

6. Do three circuits of the triceps extension exercises.

As you perform this exercise, do your best to keep your arms bent as you move them back before straightening your arms backward. If you practice your movements, they should flow into each other without any pausing. You can then use weights to increase the intensity of the exercise.

Chest press

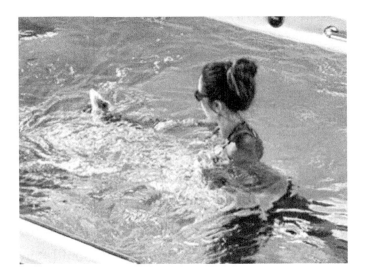

You know how important your heart health is. Therefore, you need to exercise your chest area to release all the stress and tension accumulated as the days go by.

To perform the chest press, you need to:

1. Stand straight in the shallow end, then allow your arms to rest at your sides underneath the water.

2. Open your palms and proceed to press your fingers against each other.

3. Lift your arms in front of you without bending them, then bring your hands towards each other as if you are hugging a tree.

4. Flip your palms and bring your arms back to the sides.

5. Once you are at the starting point, repeat the exercise.

As you do the chest press, you should be able to feel a stretch on your shoulder area, chest area, and arms. The stretch should be comfortable, not painful.

Pool pushups

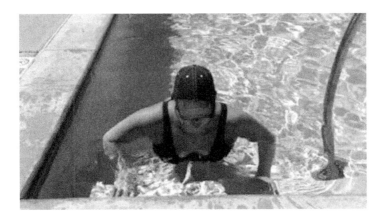

Many people are not fans of doing pushups because they lack the arm strength to do them. However, you can make your work easier by performing pool pushups.

To engage in this exercise, you should:

1. Enter the pool and move a few feet away from the wall. Your hands should be able to touch the wall when you lean forward.

2. Place your hands shoulder-width apart on the wall and align them with your legs.

3. Proceed to lean towards the wall. Your elbows should move out to the sides as you do the pushup.

4. Straighten your arms and go back to the starting position.

5. Repeat the exercise 10 times.

6. Do three circuits of the exercises.

A lot of the exercises above should not be too hard to perform. However, their repetitive nature makes for a good workout since you will exercise muscles not accustomed to it. But don't be in a hurry to do as many circuits of the exercises as possible. Instead, start with one circuit to get a feel of all the exercises, then gradually increase the number of circuits you can perform.

Chapter 4: Aerobic Exercises For Flexibility

Joint aches and muscle pain are often associated with aging. But the truth is that if you've made a habit of not stretching your body, you shouldn't be surprised when it becomes harder to move as you enter your senior years. Fortunately, you can become more flexible by doing certain exercises.

These include:

Water walking

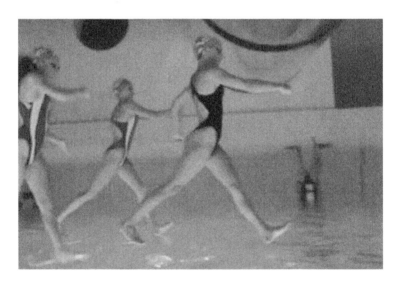

To start this series of exercises, enter the pool and stand at one end of the shallow end. Next, start walking towards the other end as you move your arms in tune with your footsteps.

Try to take larger footsteps as you walk and walk a little faster than you normally do on land.

Do this exercise for 2 to 5 minutes.

Flutter kicks

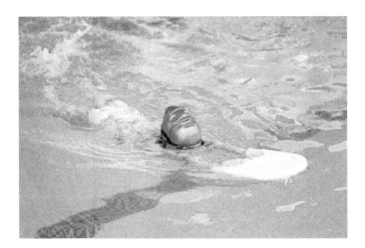

Flutter kicks are designed to propel you forward, but you can do them in place to exercise different muscles. To do this exercise, you should:

1. Grip the side of the pool as your belly faces downwards.

2. Straighten your legs behind you as far back as they can go, and keep your feet together. The aim is to lie in a straight line.

3. Kick a foot up and return it down as you kick the opposite for up. Do your best not to lower your body as you kick your feet up and down. Do not bend your knees.

4. Continue the exercise for 15 to 30 seconds.

You can hold on to a kickboard if you'd rather move about as you perform this exercise.

Leg lifts

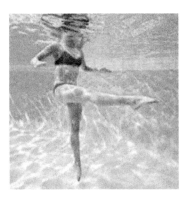

Leg lifts are a great exercise for your core, hips, and leg muscles. You need to:

1. Stand up straight and ensure that you are comfortable.

2. Proceed to lift your right leg to your side as far up as it can go, then put it down again.

3. Repeat the exercise 10 times or until you feel tired.

4. Next, lift your left leg to your side as far up as possible, then put it back down again.

5. Repeat the exercise 10 times and gradually increase the number of lifts as the days go by.

If you find it difficult to balance as you lift your leg up, you can hold on to your kickboard or the pool wall. But as your flexibility and balance improve, try to do the exercise without holding on to anything.

Leg swings

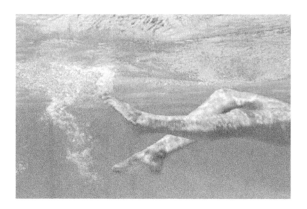

When you want to increase your flexibility, taking control of your bodily movements is important. Focus on your spatial awareness as you do leg swings.

To perform this exercise, you should:

1. Enter the pool and hold on to the edge as you face sideways.

2. Next, swing your outside leg outwards in front of you and hold the position for several seconds and then swing it backward and hold the position.

3. Repeat the exercise for several seconds and then exercise the other leg.

As you swing your legs, do not lean too much against the side of the pool. You want to improve your flexibility, which means taking steps.

Page | 50

Wall pushups

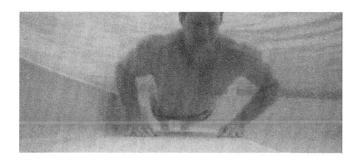

If one of your goals is to increase flexibility and build your upper body strength, you need to perform wall pushups. Due to the nature of water, you should manage to perform the exercise without putting undue stress on your joints.

To perform this exercise, you need to:

1. Stand up straight as you face the wall of the swimming pool. Place your palms on the edge of the pool.

2. Bend your elbows as you move towards the wall. Move as close to it as possible without leaning your body on it.

3. Straighten your arms as you push out, and then repeat the exercise.

4. Do ten pushups and repeat the exercise circuit twice more.

As you do wall pushups, you need to get a firm hold of your footing. You'll land in the water if you slip, but it will break your rhythm.

Arm curls

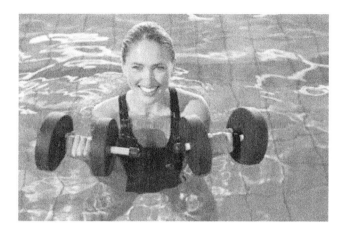

Using water weights is the best way to perform this exercise. You can use foam dumbbells.

To perform this exercise, you should:

1. Stand in the pool.

2. Place your hands by your sides and with your palms facing out. Make sure you're holding the water weights comfortably.

3. Next, bend your arms as you curl your hands upwards, then back down.

4. List your arm up and down in quick succession. The quickness of your movements will determine how effective your workout will be. The quicker you are, the more you'll be able to feel the resistance.

5. Continue with the exercise until you feel tired.

If you are not in a position to use water weights, you can still exercise without the use of weights. This will lessen the resistance you face, but you'll still be able to get some exercise in. You can always increase the intensity of the exercise later on as you get more comfortable.

Arm curls work on your wrists, elbows, and shoulders. They loosen the joints, giving you more flexibility, thus making them especially good for those who don't regularly exercise their non-dominant hand.

Arm circles

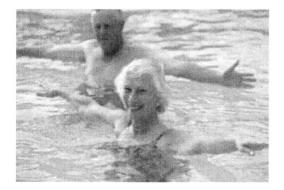

Please do this exercise in an area that will allow the water to reach your shoulders. If you are uncomfortable with going to the deep end, you can squat down in the shallow end until the water reaches your shoulder.

To perform this exercise, you should:

1. Lift your arms to your sides until they reach shoulder height. Ensure your arms are parallel to the ground and your palms are facing downwards.

2. Move your arms forward in a circular motion for 10 to 20 seconds.

3. Once the time is up, move your arms in a circular motion in the reverse direction—exercise for 10 to 20 seconds.

You may feel a pleasant strain on your arms and shoulders as you move your arms. However, you may feel uncomfortable if you have issues with your wrists. In this case, you should be careful not to move your wrists while performing the exercise.

Chest fly

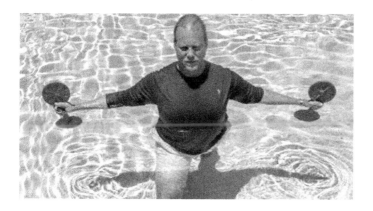

To perform this exercise, you should:

1. Place your arms in front of you with your palms facing each other and touching.

2. Next, move your arms to your sides as you push them through the water.

3. Once done, move your arms to the starting position.

4. Perform this exercise for 15 to 30 seconds.

Try to move your arms as quickly as possible as you perform the exercise. This will increase the resistance you face from the water. You can also use water weights to add resistance.

Calf raises

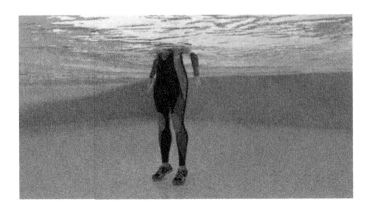

Now and then, you may find yourself reaching for something on a high shelf. For many seniors, this is a recipe for disaster as they end up straining their backs since they don't stretch regularly.

If you perform calf raises, you will manage to stretch your back in a safe environment. Plus, regular exercise will increase your flexibility and lessen the chances of injury as you go about your day-to-day life.

To perform this exercise, you should:

1. Stand near the edge of the pool.

2. Place a hand on the wall to support yourself.

3. Relax your body and shift your weight to your feet.

4. Lift your heels and hold the position for a few seconds.

5. Return to the starting position.

As you become used to the exercise, you should try to relax the hands you place on the edge of the pool.

Winding down

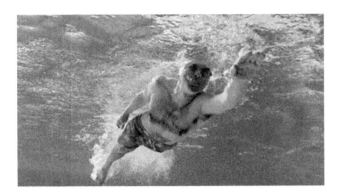

After your exercises, you should spend a few minutes cooling down. To do this, you can swim about leisurely or take a walk in the pool. Remember, water tends to shield you as you exercise, but you're still engaging your muscles and giving your body a good workout. Cooling down slowly ensures you're not sore later.

All in all:

When you want to exercise your full body and improve your flexibility, it would be good to keep in mind that you're allowed to progress bit by bit.

If you need support, use a floatation device. If you lack stamina, reduce the number of repetitions as you exercise, and if you need to challenge yourself, use weights and speed up the exercises. This way, you'll be able to achieve your goals.

Now let's look at the water exercises you can perform to increase your strength.

Chapter 5: Water Exercises For Strength

There are a few things less disheartening than having to depend on someone else to do things you could do when you were younger. But when you realize that strengthening your body can help you get your autonomy, suddenly, things don't look so grim anymore.

As they say, it's never too late to exercise your body, regain your strength and take back your life. You only need to set aside some time to perform water exercises. An exercise routine that you can use to strengthen your body is as follows:

Water walking

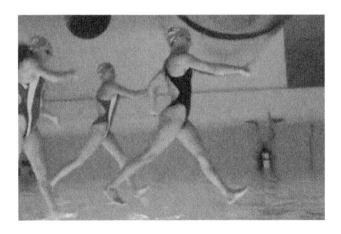

By now, you know the importance of walking in water. This exercise can work as a warmup exercise when you want to engage in other exercises and is also a full-body exercise by its merit.

But when trying to increase your strength, you should not be content with taking a leisurely walk now and then. Instead, you should shift your focus to power walking. Power walking demands you power your way through the water. You'll be swinging your arms as you walk as quickly as possible towards your target.

And once you can increase your heart rate without feeling like the world is ending, you can shift to jogging.

Targeted water marching

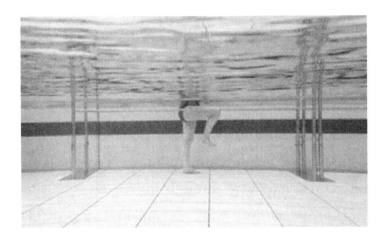

The thing with marching is that you need to pay closer attention to your body movements than you would when taking a walk. This allows you to check your posture as you try to build muscle strength.

When you march, you'll feel a pull at various parts of your body. Your thighs, abdomen, back, arms, and legs will bear most of the impact, and by marching strongly, you'll strengthen those muscles.

To perform this exercise, you should;

1. Stand in the pool in chest-deep water.

2. Place your hands at your side and make a fist.

3. Bend both arms at the elbow and ensure that your upper arms touch your sides. Ensure your biceps and triceps are engaged and tight.

4. Raise your right leg until it reaches the knee position, then raise the left leg as you lower the right leg. Keep marching in place, and ensure that you hit the ground with the ball of your feet before you allow your heels to follow.

5. As you march, move your opposite arm in tune with the opposite leg without straightening it and keep your back straight.

6. March for 15 to 45 seconds and then release the position.

Calf raises

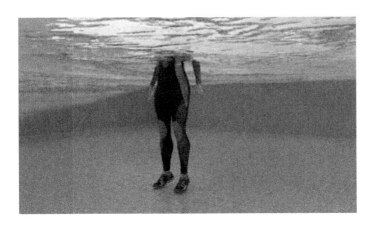

Calf raises are great for strengthening your legs and stretching your body. To perform this exercise, you need to:

1. Stand in the pool and ensure your feet are flat on the ground.

2. Allow your arms to rest by your sides and open your palms.

3. Keep your fingers close together and your hands straight down.

4. Slowly proceed to raise your heels until you stand on your toes.

5. Hold the position for about 1 to 2 seconds.

6. Slowly return to the starting position.

7. Repeat the exercise for several seconds.

As you perform this exercise, be gentle and move slowly whenever you raise yourself and come down again. Your feet play the important role of supporting your body weight, and you don't want to hurt them even as you try to strengthen them.

Bended knee chest fly

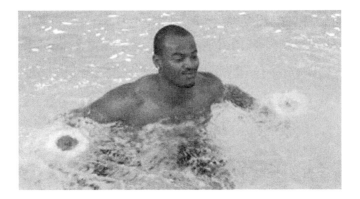

It's always important to exercise our chest muscles since you need them to function properly to perform a variety of movements.

To perform this exercise, you should:

1. Place the right foot in front of your left foot and proceed to bend your knees. Your neck and head should be above the water, but your shoulders should be submerged.

2. Lift your arms out to make a T-shape, and ensure your elbows are straight.

3. Imitate a pushing motion as you move your arms towards each other in front of you. Allow your palms to touch.

4. Flip your hands so that the back of your palms touch, then slowly move your arms back to the T-shape position. Your reverse movements should resemble a pulling motion.

5. Pause for 1 to 2 seconds and then repeat the exercise.

6. Repeat the exercise 10 times.

As you do the chest fly, you should be able to feel your movements and control them. Do not allow the water to sway you or pull you along. Push against it if you have to.

Sideways bicep curls

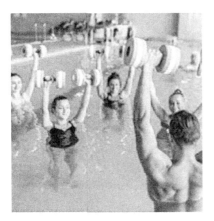

To do this exercise, you should:

- Head to a pool part that allows the water to reach your shoulders.

- Spread your legs so they are shoulder-width apart, and keep them straight.

- Extend your arms to your sides and keep them straight.

- Slowly bend your elbows such that your arms are at 90 degrees. You should be able to feel a pull as you do this exercise. If you don't, tighten your biceps.

- Hold the position, then straighten your forearms to stand in a T-shape position.

- Perform 10 to 12 repetitions of the exercise.

If you wish to increase the intensity of the exercise, you can make a fist with your hands. You can also cup the water with your fingers as you move your hands.

Arm raises

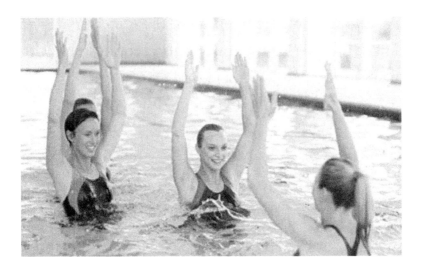

To do this exercise, stand in the pool with your shoulders submerged in the water.

1. Once you're in position, carefully stand with your legs shoulder-width apart.

2. Allow your arms to rest at your sides. That is your starting position.

3. Next, lift your arms slowly at your sides, and do not bend your elbows. Your arms should rest just underneath the water.

4. Picture yourself pressing the water down as you return your hands to the starting position.

5. Repeat the exercise 10 to 12 times.

6. Flip your palms in the opposite direction and raise them up until they're just underneath the water.

7. Hold the position for 1 second, and then press down slowly until your hands return to the starting position.

8. Repeat the exercise 10 to 12 times.

The trick to doing this exercise is to imagine the water as a hard surface. Press down as hard as possible to create more room. If you keep your hands straight, you'll feel greater resistance as you push down. As you push up, picture yourself pushing against a hard surface for added resistance.

Wall pushups

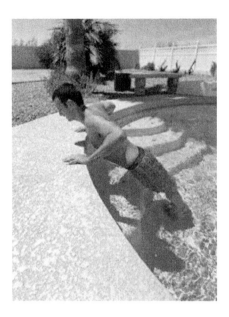

You can do this exercise at the shallow end of the pool. To do it, you should:

1. Stand with your hands on the wall of the pool. They should be shoulder width apart or more.

2. Plant your feet firmly on the ground and lean towards the wall.

3. Push back to the starting position, all while taking care not to lose your balance.

4. Repeat the exercise 10 times.

As you become more comfortable with wall pushups, you should try to repeat the exercise circuit 2 to 3 times. Once a circuit is complete, rest for 30 seconds before you start the next circuit.

Hip flexion

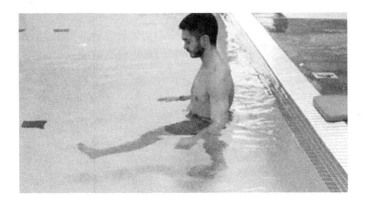

Before you perform this exercise, move next to the stair railing or the pool wall. And then:

1. Stand with your feet shoulder-width apart, then place your right hand on the stair railing or the pull wall.

2. Keep your eyes looking forward and your back straight. Keep your knee locked to prevent it from bending.

3. Swing your right leg slowly, fast as possible, then swing it backward.

4. Repeat the exercise 10 times.

5. Once done, turn around and exercise the other leg.

As you do this exercise, you can make it more interesting by pointing your toes whenever you move your leg forward and flexing your feet when you move your legs back. Remember, you're trying to strengthen your body, and your toes and feet need strengthening too.

Hip adduction

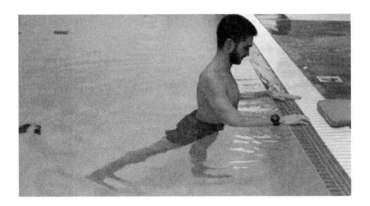

To do this exercise, you should:

1. Move to the side of the pool or stand next to the railing.

2. While holding the railing with your right hand, raise your leg out towards the side.

3. Bring your left leg backward and keep your toes forward. Do not bend your knee.

4. Repeat the exercise 10 times.

5. Once done, turn and hold the railing with your left hand.

6. Swing your right leg in front of you without bending your knee, then move it backward.

7. Repeat the exercise 10 times.

As you perform this exercise, you should always point your toes forward and keep your knees tight, even when moving your legs backward.

Hamstring curls

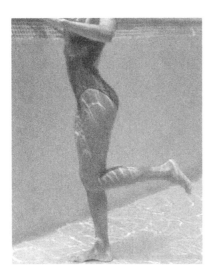

To perform this exercise, you need to:

1. Stand up straight inside the pool. You can face the wall and hold it with your hand or both hands if you desire extra balance.

2. Bend your knee as you move your leg back towards your glutes.

3. Move your foot back down without moving the opposite hip.

4. Repeat the exercise 10 times and then switch to the other leg.

As you do this exercise, you may notice a tendency to move your opposite hip slightly as you bring the other leg down. If you do so, you may feel a slight pain in the hip, which is not ideal. Train yourself to move your leg without shifting your hip.

Flutter kicks

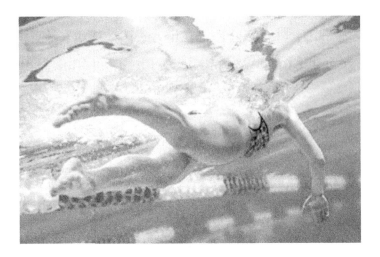

To do this exercise, you should:

1. Stretch your hands back to hold on to the wall as your belly faces downwards. Your feet should drift behind you.

2. Straighten your legs, then proceed to kick your feet up and down.

3. Perform the exercise for 15 to 30 seconds.

This type of exercise will help you strengthen your legs and feet. Do not bend your knees as you do it.

Wall chair

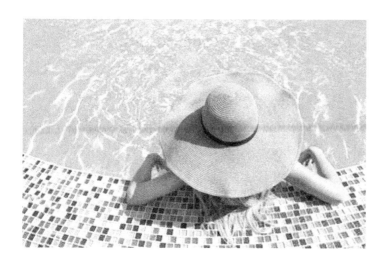

This exercise will test your flexibility, but it is great for strengthening your body. To do it, you need to:

1. Stand against the pool wall. Your back should touch the wall, and your hands should reach out to hold the wall. You can extend your arms over your shoulders in an effort to grasp the wall.

2. Once comfortable, lift your feet up as you bring your knees towards your chest.

3. Hold for 5 to 10 seconds, then put your feet back down.

4. Repeat the exercise 10 times.

As you enter your senior years, it is vital to remember that your body should not be in pain just because you've moved a certain way. You can exercise to strengthen it and increase your flexibility. And although you don't need special equipment to strengthen your body, you may want to look into exercise equipment such as flippers, hand paddles, water weights, and pool noodles if you wish to increase the intensity of your workouts.

Now that you know what to do to strengthen your body, let's look at full-body exercises capable of helping you turn the heat up.

Chapter 6: Holistic Aerobic Workouts

There are many advantages to giving yourself a full-body workout whenever you exercise in the pool. Even so, it's in your best interest to step up things a little bit to get the most out of your workouts. The following exercise routine will help you do so:

All-round walking

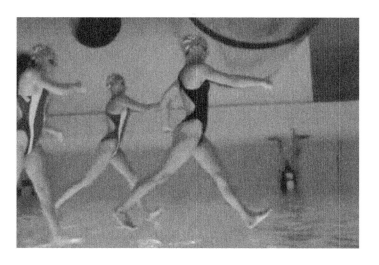

For this exercise, you need to stand in the pool. The water should be waist or chest-deep.

1. Once in position, walk 10 to 20 steps forward and then 10 to 20 steps backward. Try to walk as fast as possible to increase the difficulty.

2. Next, jog for 30 seconds. You should jog in place instead of moving across the pool to avoid the water pushing you along.

3. Walk in place for 30 seconds.

4. Once done, walk sideways for 20 steps, then change directions and walk 20 steps in the opposite direction.

You can increase the intensity of the exercise by holding your kickboard vertically as you walk in the water. Ensure that your kickboard is underneath the water so that the water can offer added resistance.

Forward and side lunges

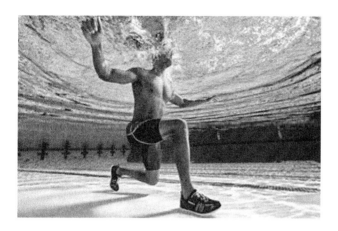

For this exercise, you should:

1. Stand near the pool wall. Doing this will allow you to hold it for support if needed.

2. Once you're in place, take a large step forward with your right leg. Your knee should bend, but it should not advance past your toes.

3. Go back to the starting point and then move your left leg forward in a similar fashion.

4. Repeat the exercise 10 times and do three sets of the lunges.

5. Once done with the forward lunges, take a big step to your side with your toes facing forward and your knee bent.

6. Shift to the opposite leg and repeat the exercise.

7. Do three sets, each consisting of 10 side lunges.

You can make the lunges more interesting by walking across the pool instead of exercising in place. To do this, you will need to move one foot in front of the other as you do the lunges. Ensure you have a firm footing before performing the exercises and that you don't waste time between the movements.

Balance stand

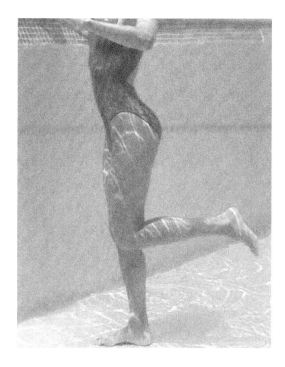

For this exercise, you should:

1. Stand on your right leg.

2. Raise your left leg to your hip level.

3. If you have a pool noodle, place it under the raised leg as you hold it with both hands.

4. Hold the position for 30 seconds.

5. Switch positions and stand on your left leg as you raise your right leg.

6. Hold the position for 30 seconds.

7. Do 2 to 5 sets of the exercise.

If you find it difficult to use a pool noodle, you can do the exercise without holding onto it. You can hold onto the poolside if you wish for extra support.

Sidestepping

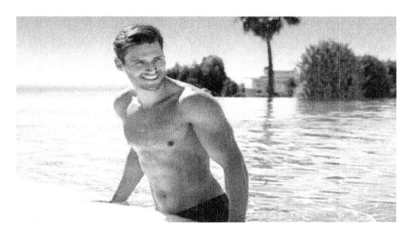

For this exercise, you should:

1. Stand up straight while facing the pool wall.

2. Start walking sideways with your toes and body still facing the wall. Take 10 to 20 steps sideways, bringing your left leg towards your right leg.

3. Change directions and bring your right leg towards your left leg. Take 10 to 20 steps.

4. Repeat the set twice.

As you do this exercise, you need to check your posture. You should move in a straight line and keep your legs straight. Do not try to cross your legs as you move.

Hip kicks

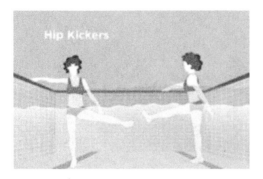

For this exercise, you should:

1. Stand in the pool next to the pool wall.

2. Move your right leg forward as if you are kicking a ball. As you kick, keep your knee straight instead of bending it.

3. Return to the starting point.

4. Move your right leg to the side. Mimic the kicking action without bending your knee.

5. Go to the starting position and then kick the keg back.

6. Next, move your left leg forward as if kicking a ball. Do not bend your knee as you kick.

7. Return the leg to the starting position.

8. Move your left leg to your side but do not bend your knee as you kick.

9. Return to o the starting position, then kick to the back without moving your knee.

10. Repeat the exercise 10 times and proceed to do three sets of the exercise.

The trick to doing this exercise is staying near the pool wall in case you need support but far enough to safely kick your leg backward without hitting the wall. Also, do not be too enthusiastic as you kick because doing so may cause you to slip and lose your balance.

Pool planks

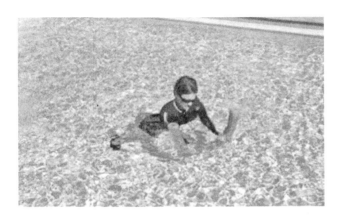

For this exercise, you should:

1. Hold on to a pool noodle. Your hands should be shoulder-width apart, and the noodle should be parallel to the pool floor.

2. Lean forward and submerge the pool noodle in the water until it reaches the bottom. Your elbows should straighten, but your toes should remain planted on the pool floor.

3. Keep your body straight and hold for 15 to 60 seconds.

4. Repeat the exercise 3 to 5 times.

The pool noodle helps you sink downwards as you do the pool plank, but it is possible to do the plank without using it.

But you can also use water weights to make it easier to sink down and harder to come back up.

Deep water bicycle

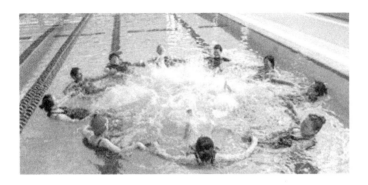

For this exercise, you should:

1. Stand in deep water and place a pool noodle or two behind you. Your arms should rest on top of the noodle.

2. Proceed to move your legs in a cycling motion.

3. Exercise for 3 to 5 minutes.

If you are not comfortable balancing on a pool noodle, you can move to the pool wall and rest your arms there as you perform this exercise. The idea is to exercise the lower part of the body even as you give your upper body a slight workout.

Arm raises

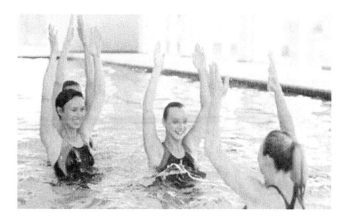

For this exercise, you should:

1. Stand in the pool. The water should be able to able to cover your shoulders. You should also use resistance gloves or arm paddles for added resistance.

2. Straighten your arms to your sides and then form 90 degrees angles. At this point, your hands should remain submerged in the water. Keep your shoulders relaxed and down.

3. Next, raise your arms up toward the surface of the water and then return them to your sides.

4. Repeat the exercise 10 times.

5. Do 3 sets of the exercise.

Do not forget to straighten your hands to your sides after each arm raise. That extra step is vital as it allows you to exercise your upper arms as you raise them to bend your elbows.

Also, if you want to make the exercise more intense, you can do it as you balance on one leg. But if you choose to do this, you should plan to interchange the raised leg instead of balancing on one leg for the entire exercise.

Pushups

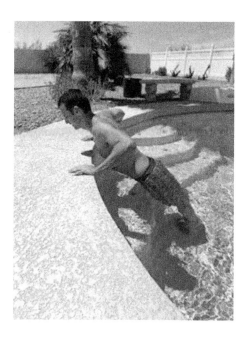

For this exercise, you should:

1. Stand in the pool and move back so you can straighten your arms and place your hands shoulder-width apart on the pool's edge.

2. Plant your feet on the pool floor and keep your body straight as you lean towards the pool edge. Do not lean your chest on the pool's edge.

3. Next, straighten up by pressing your weight with your hands.

4. Repeat the exercise 10 times.

5. Do three sets of this exercise.

If you wish, you can hold the position for a few seconds once you are halfway on your way back. If you do this, you will be able to feel a greater burn.

Standing knee lift

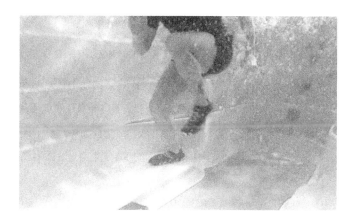

For this exercise, you should:

1. Stand in the pool with your back touching the pool wall. Your feet should touch the floor of the pool.

2. Stand on your right leg; bend your left leg at the knee and keep the knee aligned with your left hip.

3. Perform the exercise 10 times.

4. Stand on your left leg. Your right leg should bend at the knee, and keep your knee aligned with your right hip.

5. Perform the exercise 10 times.

6. Do three sets of this exercise.

You can enhance this exercise by moving away from the wall as you perform it. But be careful not to lose your balance.

Holistic workouts work on your muscle strength and endurance. But they are not complete without you watching what you eat, having a healthy sleep routine, and working on your emotional well-being. Thus, you should plan to work on all aspects of your life to benefit fully from a holistic lifestyle.

Now let's focus on exercises you can perform when you want to really challenge your body.

Chapter 7: Advanced Aerobics Workouts

Rarely do we consider exercise fun, but it can be when you find new and exciting ways to exercise. Some exercises you can do to spice up your workouts include:

Triceps dip

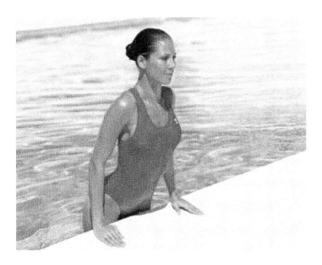

For this exercise, you should:

1. Move to the pool and place your back on the pool wall, with your feet in the water. Your hands should be at your sides, gripping the edge.

2. Proceed to move your body downwards and allow your elbow to bend until your arms form 90 degrees angles.

3. Straighten back up as you push through your hands.

4. Do 15 reps of the exercise.

This exercise works your core and triceps. But you should be able to feel a burn on your shoulder area and thighs.

Incline pushup

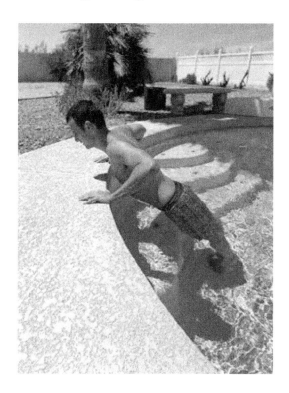

For this exercise, you should:

1. Face the pool wall and move back a bit so you can touch the pool's edge with your hands, even as you keep your body inclined.

2. Place your hands shoulder-width apart on the pool edge. Make sure that your arms and legs are straight. Your body should be able to form a straight line.

3. Proceed to lean towards the pool wall until your elbows bend at 90 degrees. Your chest should be near the edge of the pool.

4. Move back up until your arms are straight again. This counts for one rep.

5. Perform the exercise 10 to 12 times.

Remember to be careful when doing pool pushups since slipping will knock you off your balance.

Jumping jack

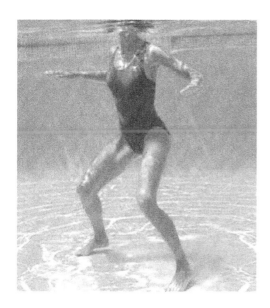

For this exercise, you should:

1. Stand in the pool with your feet hip-width apart. Place your arms at your sides.

2. Raise your arms to your sides and up to touch over your head as you move your feet more than shoulder-width apart.

3. Move your hands back down as you bring your legs together and count that as one rep.

4. Jump 20 times without pausing.

Jumping jacks can get interesting when you're in the pool since you will be working against the water and splashing it about. The important part is keeping your rhythm and balance as you work your shoulders, upper back, quads, and glutes.

Squat jump

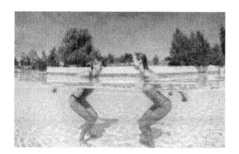

For this exercise, you should:

1. Stand in the pool and ensure the water comes up to your shoulders when you squat.

2. Stand with your feet hip-width apart and your hands at your sides.

3. Bend your knees in a squat as you bring your hands together in a prayer position.

4. Jump up as you return your arms to your sides. That is one rep.

5. Perform 10 to 12 squat jumps.

As you perform this exercise, you should aim to jump explosively off the floor before returning to a squatting position. This exercise engages your core, calves, hamstrings, glutes, and quads.

Mountain climbers

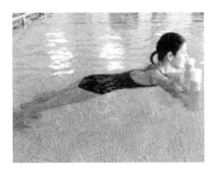

For this exercise, you should:

1. Get into the plank position. Your palms should touch the floor, and your body should remain inclined as your toes touch the floor behind you. Try to keep your body as straight as possible.

2. Next, move your right knee forward until it almost touches your right elbow, and then move your left knee forward towards your left elbow quickly. Count that as one rep.

3. Perform the exercise 15 times.

Mountain climbers are quite challenging even though they are easier on your core when you do them in water. But once you are comfortable in the squat position, you can train yourself to move your legs as you do the mountain climber.

Ideally, you'd want to perform the exercise fast, but there is no shame in starting off slow.

Tuck jump

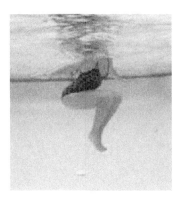

For this exercise, you should:

1. Stand in the pool with your feet hip-width apart. Place your arms at your sides.

2. Proceed to bend your knees slightly as you raise your arms to shoulder height with your elbows bent. Your palms should face downwards.

3. Bend deep, shoot up as you jump, and allow your knees to touch your open palms.

4. Move back down with your knees bent and straighten up with your arms back at your sides. That is one rep.

5. Perform the exercise 10 times.

The tuck jump is a high-intensity move that works on your full body. Thus, you must exercise proper form and work on your movements to make them as smooth as possible.

Scissors kick

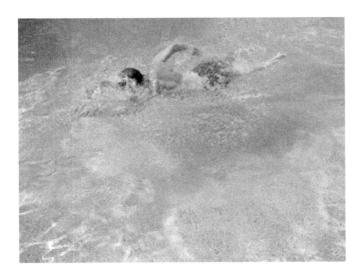

For this exercise, you should:

1. Lean against the pool wall, with your arms out wide as you hold on to the pool's edge. Ensure your body is straight.

2. Proceed to lift your feet off the floor.

3. Kick your feet up and down with your toes pointed. Count every two kicks as one rep.

4. Perform the exercise 15 times.

This exercise works on your glutes, thighs, and core. But it may be uncomfortable to reach overhead to support yourself by holding on to the wall. Focus on your abs as you do the exercise to keep your mind occupied.

Knee lift

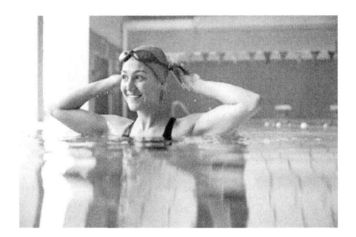

For this exercise, you should:

1. Stand in the pool with the feet more than hip-width apart.

2. Bend your arms and then place them behind your head.

3. Lift your right knee towards your right elbow and your left knee towards the left elbow. You can count that as one rep.

4. Perform 10 to 12 repetitions.

As you do this exercise, picture yourself pushing down even as you lift your legs up through the water. This will create greater resistance.

Reverse fly

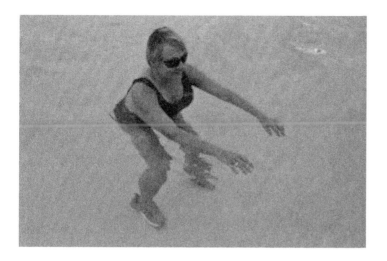

For this exercise, you should:

1. Stand up with your feet hip-width apart.

2. Bend your knees slightly, then bend your body at the waist.

3. Make a fist with both your hands and allow them to touch downwards.

4. Lift both hands to your sides until they are at shoulder length. Squeeze your shoulders as you lift your hands.

5. Return your fists down past your knees. Count that as one rep.

6. Perform the exercise 15 times.

This exercise works on your quads, glutes, core, and upper back. If you place your shoulders and hands in the water, you will face stronger resistance as you work those muscles.

Lateral lunge

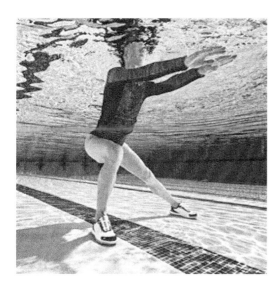

For this exercise, you should:

1. Stand up straight with your feet hip-width apart. Place your hands by your sides.

2. Step to the right as wide as you can. Your left leg should straighten even as your right knee bends with the toes facing frontward. Try forming a 90-degree angle with your bended knee.

3. Push back up as you lift the right knee until it is near your chest. Both your hands should be around the knee.

4. Return to the starting position and count that as one rep.

5. Perform the exercise 10 times and then change sides.

Lateral lunges are great at working your quads, core, glues, and hamstrings. The water helps make it easier and helps you work on your balance as you perform the exercises.

All in all, this exercise routine may seem more difficult than the previous routines simply due to how the exercises are, but the high-intensity exercises are still low-impact. This means they won't be tough on your body.

The important thing is to get the exercise right so you can do it as quickly as possible for maximum impact.

Now let's look at full-body exercises that can help you build endurance.

Chapter 8: Endurance Aerobic Exercises

Endurance is something we could all use more of as we grow older. It is a quality that enables you to carry on and push your body further even when you're faced with things such as fatigue and reduced energy. To increase endurance, you can perform certain aerobic exercises. These include:

Flutter kicks

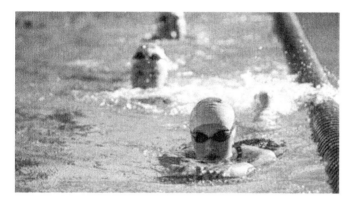

For this exercise, you should:

1. Stand tall in the pool and place your hands on the pool edge.

2. Kick your legs, one leg after the other, as you keep your legs tight, kick as hard as possible, and keep your hands straight as they hold on to the wall. Ensure your

toes point forward. You can turn them slightly inward if you wish.

3. Perform 50 to 100 kicks.

As you start, do so slowly, then increase your kicking speed as you go. Also, remember to keep your body straight, especially if you are used to slouching. The more you exercise, the more you'll be conscious of your posture, which will help you make positive changes.

Water jogging

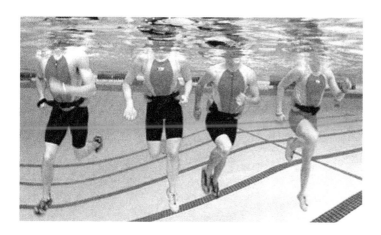

For this exercise, you should:

1. Head over to the shallow end of the pool.

2. .Start jogging across the pool, taking long strides and ensuring that your heel hits the flour before your toes. Your arms should be moving in tune with your strides. If you are not comfortable with jogging, you can take a walk.

3. Exercise for 10 minutes.

As you jog or walk, you should keep your back straight. Check your posture occasionally since you may start slouching as you get tired.

Kickboard swim

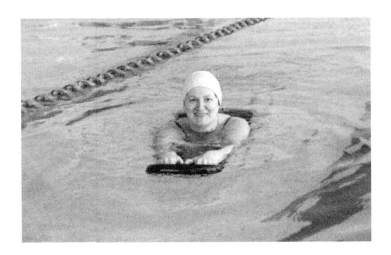

For this exercise, you should:

1. Hold on to your kickboard and extend your body behind you in a straight line.

2. Kick your legs strongly as you move across the pool. Make sure that your hands are straight as you kick your legs.

3. Kick for two to four pool lengths.

If you are not a good swimmer, you can hold on to the pool wall and kick in place. But try to keep your body straight even as you do so.

Jumping jacks

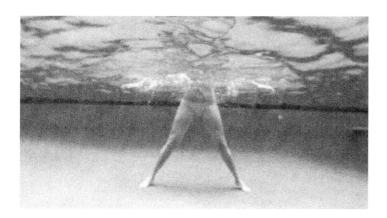

Jumping jacks used to be fun when you were younger. But as you grow older, you quickly discover that they can be quite uncomfortable to perform, especially if you suffer from aches and pains or have put on quite a bit of weight. Fortunately, you can perform them on water.

For this exercise, you should:

1. Stand up straight in the pool and keep your feet hip-width apart. Place your arms at your sides.

2. Proceed to raise your arms horizontally and then raise them over your head, even as you jump up and spread your feet to the sides.

3. Bring your arms back down as you bring your legs hip-width apart.

4. Do 15 to 20 jumps.

If you want stronger resistance, you can do the jumps in shoulder-deep water. This way, both your arms and feet will face resistance. You can also use ankle weights and wrist weights to make the exercise more difficult to perform.

Resisted flutter kicks

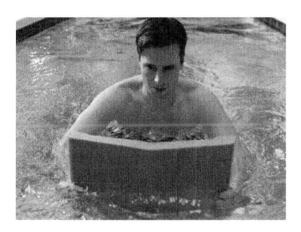

For this exercise, you should:

1. Get your kickboard and place your hands at the bottom of it. Your kickboard should be standing in a vertical position.

2. Proceed to extend your body on the water's surface. Your body should be in a straight line.

3. Kick your legs, one after the other, keep the kicks strong, and ensure that you keep your toes pointed inwards. As you kick, ensure that your hands remain straight, even as you continue holding the kickboard.

4. Kick for 2 to 4 pool lengths.

Using a kickboard allows you to perform this exercise even if you are not a strong swimmer. However, you can stick to kicking across the shallow end if you are not comfortable with heading to the deep end of the pool.

Pool burpee

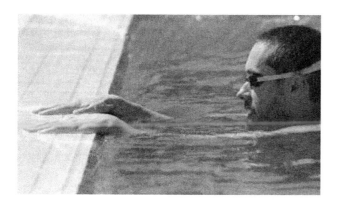

For this exercise, you should:

1. Move near the pool wall and use your hands to grip the edge.

2. Allow your body to drift behind you in a straight line.

3. Move your right knee towards your chest, then quickly move your left knee towards your chest.

4. Alternate moving your lengths and perform the exercise 20 to 40 times.

Moving as quickly as possible will help you get the most out of this exercise. You can also add ankle weights to make the exercise more challenging.

Tuck jumps

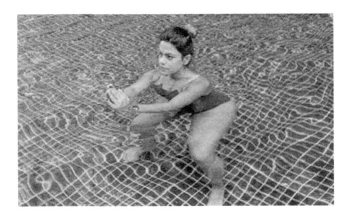

For this exercise, you should:

1. Stand up in the pool with your feet hip-width apart in waist-deep or chest-deep water.

2. Slightly bend your knees, lift your arms to your sides, and bend your hands downwards. Your palms should face down.

3. Bend your legs a little more, then jump up, so your knees move towards your palms. The idea is to try and use your knees to touch your hands.

4. Perform the exercise 10 to 15 times.

This exercise exercises your muscles, but it also does an important job of improving your balance. If you can't jump as high as you want, jump as high as you can, even as you check your posture. Over time, you will manage to jump higher.

Hacky sack

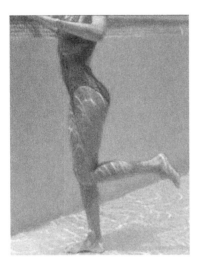

This exercise challenges your timing and balance. It's a good thing it is done in a pool as this allows you to fail many times as you try to get the exercise right.

For this exercise, you should:

1. Stand up in chest-deep water.

2. Lift your right leg and keep your knee bent.

3. Proceed to rotate your hip as you move your foot up and inward.

4. Next, reach down with your left hand and touch your right foot.

5. Once done, lift your left leg with your knee bent.

6. Proceed to rotate your hip as you move your foot up and inward.

7. Reach down with your right hand and proceed to touch your left foot. Count that as one rep.

8. Perform 20 to 30 reps.

As you jump up, your lifted leg and the hand reaching out to touch it should be in a diagonal position. However, avoid bending your back as you try to reach your foot.

Ski motion

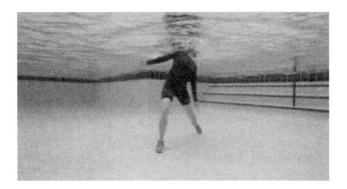

If you've always admired skiers, this is your chance to emulate their motions even if you don't get the full experience.

For this exercise, you should:

1. Stand in the pool in chest-deep water. Place your feet together.

2. Jump up and move one foot in front and one foot back.

3. Switch legs quickly as you scissor them back and forth.

4. Perform 15 to 20 reps.

As you do this exercise, you may need to balance yourself by spreading your arms straight on either side of your body.

Frog jump

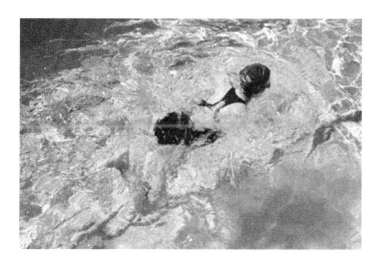

Frog jumps are a bit challenging to do on land, especially if you cannot land softly. Also, you cannot imitate the motions closely since you may end up landing on your face. But you can do them in water without worrying too much about how you land.

For this exercise, you should:

1. Stand up in chest-deep water and keep your hands at your sides and your feet together.

2. Bend your knees and jump as you move your feet to touch together at the toes. At the same time, move your hands to touch your toes.

3. Perform 15 to 20 jumps.

If you've ever seen a frog jumping, you'll have fun as you try to imitate its motion. This exercise is a bit challenging but great at exercising your body and improving your balance and coordination.

As you know, various exercise combinations can create a full-body workout. You can start with simple combinations if you're new to water exercises and gradually try high-intensity exercises. You can greatly increase the impact of the exercises you do by increasing your speed and using various equipment to increase resistance. With patience and consistency, you can be sure to get in the full body workout that works wonders for your mind and body.

Conclusion

As you grow older, you need to think of the best way to exercise to achieve the best results. Water aerobics has proven capable of providing such results because it creates a comfortable environment for you to perform a wide range of movements without the cages and pains that come from land-based exercises.

To start water exercises, you only need to get the right gear, learn some exercises and set some time to exercise at least 3 to 5 days a week. If you do this, you'll soon see some encouraging results as your physical and mental well-being improve.

PS: I'd like your feedback. If you are happy with this book, please leave a review on Amazon.

Please leave a review for this book on Amazon by visiting the page below:

https://amzn.to/2VMR5qr

Printed in Great Britain
by Amazon